Making Y Hand Sa

— — — — — ❧❧❧❧ — — — —

Protect Yourself Against The Virus – How To Make 500 Ml. Of Hand Sanitizer In Just 25 Minutes!

By Health's First Products & Samantha Johnson

1

(including but not limited to your doctor, attorney, financial advisor or such other professional advisor) before using any of the suggested remedies, techniques, or information in this book.

Upon using the contents and information contained in this book, you agree to hold harmless the Author from and against any damages, costs, and expenses, including any legal fees potentially resulting from the application of any of the information provided by this book. This disclaimer applies to any loss, damages or injury caused by the use and application, whether directly or indirectly, of any advice or information presented, whether for breach of contract, tort, negligence, personal injury, criminal intent, or under any other cause of action.

You agree to accept all risks of using the information presented inside this book.

You agree that by continuing to read this book, where appropriate and/or necessary, you shall consult a professional (including but not limited to your doctor, attorney, or financial advisor or such other advisor as needed) before using any of the suggested remedies, techniques, or information in this book.

Table of Contents

Introduction

Hands, if or not ungloved, are among the chief methods of spreading disease or for moving bacterial contamination. The usage of hand disinfectants is a part of the procedure for fantastic pollution control for employees working in hospital surroundings, or people involved with aseptic processing and inside cleanrooms. Even though there are lots of distinct sorts of hand sanitizers accessible that there are differences using their efficacy, and many don't match the European standard available sanitization.

Employees operating in hospitals and cleanrooms take various kinds of microorganisms in their palms, and these germs can be easily transferred from person to person or by individual to gear or surfaces that are critical. For critical surgeries, some security is given by sporting gloves. However, gloves aren't appropriate for many gloves and activities or even frequently sanitized or, if they're of an improper layout, can pick up and move contamination.

Hence, the sanitization of palms (either gloved or ungloved) is an equally significant part contamination management in hospitals, to steer clear of staff-to-patient cross-contamination or before undertaking surgical or clinical procedures; and also, for aseptic trainings such as the dispensing of medications. Additionally, not only is that the usage of a hand sanitizer required before undertaking these programs, it's likewise essential that the sanitizer is good at removing a large population of germs. Various studies have revealed that when a very low number of germs persist following the use of a sanitizer; subsequently, the subpopulation can grow, which can be resistant to potential programs.

There are lots of commercially available hand sanitizers having the most frequently used forms being alcohol-based fluids or dyes. Much like other varieties of disinfectants, hand sanitizers are effective against different germs based upon their style of action. Together with the most typical alcohol-based hand sanitizers, the manner of activity contributes to bacterial cell passing through cytoplasm leakage, denaturation of protein, and ultimate cell lysis (alcohols are among those so-called 'membrane disrupters'). The benefits of using alcohols as hand sanitizers incorporate a comparatively low price, small odor, and a fast evaporation (restricted residual activity contributes to shorter contact times). Additionally, alcohols have an established cleansing activity.

In picking a hands sanitizer, the pharmaceutical business or clinic will have to think about whether the program will be forced into human skin to gloved hands or to either, and if it's necessary to become sporicidal. Hand sanitizers fall into two different classes: alcohol established, which can be more prevalent, and also non-alcohol based. Such factors affect both upon price as well as the health and security of the employees utilizing the hand sanitizer because most generally accessible alcohol-based sanitizers may lead to excessive drying of the skin; and also a few non-alcohols established sanitizers may be irritating to skin. Alcohol hand sanitizers are intended to prevent irritation through owning sterile properties (color and odor-free) and components that manage skin protection and attention via re-fatting agents.

Alcohols have a lengthy history of usage as disinfectants as a result of inherent antiseptic properties from bacteria and some viruses. To succeed, some water must be blended with alcohol to apply effect against germs, together with the very best variety falling between 60 and 95 percent (most industrial hand sanitizers are approximately 70 percent). The most widely used alcohol-based hand sanitizers have been Isopropyl alcohol or some type of denatured ethanol (for instance, Industrial Methylated Spirits). The more prevalent non-alcohol established sanitizers include either chlorhexidine or hexachlorophene. Additives may also be contained in hand sanitizers so as to grow the anti-inflammatory properties.

Chapter 1: Does Hand Sanitizers Work Against Viruses?

Before offering recipes for making natural antibacterial gel, we want to clarify what its properties are. This type of gels has antibacterial properties, so they kill a variety of bacteria they also have fungicidal properties, that is, they eliminate pathogenic fungi, and they are also powerful disinfectants, eliminating a wide variety of germs. But what about viruses?

As indicated by the WHO, antibacterial gels are not suitable against viruses, as they are bactericidal and not virucidal; just like with antibiotic drugs, they fight against bacteria, not against viruses. However, there are some disinfecting gels with a virucidal effect, and in this case, it is indicated on the product label.

Wash your hands thoroughly as indicated, you should start by using soap and water and then apply the gel to both hands thoroughly (both palms and backs and between fingers) and let it dry. The part of hand washing should last between 40 and 60 seconds and that of hand disinfection between 20 and 30 seconds. You should never use only gel; except you've washed with soap and water for a very short time or in places and situations where there is not good access to soap and water).

Using hand sanitizers by those that have a great deal of touch with the general public, together with regular hand washing machine, would really prevent illness. The practice is straightforward. Hand sanitizers include alcohol at a concentrated form. Alcohol kills germs. Microorganisms cause illness.

Among our major concerns within our wellbeing and retaining us emptiness of germs and fungal disease would be with the support of hand sanitizer dispensers. Considering all the mortal diseases and pandemics that we've struck previously, it's quite vital for all of us to remain secure and take care of the cleanliness of ourselves and our environment, not only on which our eyes can observe, but those who we can't.

In our everyday lives, we ought to know about where the contamination and spread of virus will be possible. Crowded and often seen places such as metro stations and other people are all sources of these germs which you might even choose home. It's then important to get a convenient hand sanitizer dispenser on your luggage when traveling. In case you've got enough opportunity to clean your hands if you visit a comfortable space, do this. This will also assist in protecting yourself from germs which you may get. When a hand sanitizer is offered at precisely the exact same rest space, avail yourself of this privilege.

Often handed down, things like coins and invoices are passed around can attract viruses. This cart that you have been pushing around the supermarket, the doorway from the diner, or the countertop at the lender could all have been managed with many people who you can not tell, which got you contaminated. It's then important to guard yourself in them being moved to you by massaging your hands after each managing.

Composition of Hand Sanitizers

In order to prepare hand sanitizers at home, it is important to know the basic ingredients that are required to make it effective against the germs. Hand sanitizers are 90 percent alcohol, and about ten percent of the other ingredients that are used to add color, scent, and texture. Hand sanitizers vary in forms, some are prepared as clear gel-like liquids, and some are foamy in appearance.

Chapter 2: Basic Ingredients Required to Make a Hand Sanitizer

Irrespective of the recipe used, the following are the basic ingredients and things that you will need to make a good hand sanitizer.

These ingredients are commonly available at the medical stores or you can also find them in the super stores under the label of different companies. It is important consider the percentages of the alcohol used.

99.9% isopropyl alcohol: Rubbing alcohol and simple alcohol is used to make the base of the sanitizer. Keep the rubbing alcohol stored in a sealed and tight container, then use only when all other ingredients of the hand sanitizer are ready to combine.

98% aloe Vera gel: To get a gel-like consistency, nothing works better than aloe Vera gel. You can either use fresh gel, directly extracted from the Aloe Vera leaves or the gel that is available in the market. Aloe Vera naturally has healing properties, and it is also great for the skin.

10 % Witch hazel: Liquid extracted from witch hazel plants and is used for its disinfectant properties. The liquid contains tannins that repair skin, heal wounds, and fight bacteria.

Drops of essential oils: Essential oils are basically added to give a particular fragrance to the sanitizer. You can use any one of the following essential oils and add only a few drops to each bottle of sanitizer:

Aromatherapy Add-ons

With all of the options that you have been given above, you should feel well-prepared to make your own hand sanitizer if need be. Whether the stores are all sold out or you simply want to switch to a homemade option, all of these recipes are simple to create. There are countless essential oil options for you to use to put a creative twist on any sanitizer that is plain or relatively unscented. The following guide can assist you when you are selecting your additional ingredients.

Cinnamon

Not only is it a delicious scent that most people enjoy, but cinnamon is also known to be effective at reducing drowsiness. This invigorating scent can be added to your hand sanitizer blends for an additional boost. It is also known for helping you stay focused, a great addition for hand sanitizer that you plan on bringing with you to work. If you are prone to headaches, the scent has also been known to relieve them. It is one of the most healing essential oils out there, for good reason.

Lavender

This scent has the opposite effects of cinnamon. Lavender oil is best known for its relaxing and calming properties. People enjoy this scent when they are trying to relax or stay calm. If you plan on keeping hand sanitizer on your bedside table, making a blend with lavender essential oil would be a great decision. This is also a great scent to use if you are making hand sanitizer for your children. Because it is not so harsh, kids also generally enjoy the smell while receiving the same calming effects.

Lemon

Lemon oil is another aromatherapy option that will leave you feeling rejuvenated and energized. It is a scent that most people enjoy in the morning because it is very fresh. Many individuals will make lemon-scented hand sanitizer that is kept in the kitchen. If you are feeling down or stressed, lemon oil can help you by easing these symptoms. Overall, it is a very beneficial scent that is also very familiar to most people. Because it is so potent, you won't need to use a lot of oil to achieve all of the benefits that it has to offer.

Peppermint

Best known for calming your nerves, peppermint is a relaxing scent that most people associate with the holidays. Because of its benefits, you can use it year-round. When you add peppermint oil to your hand sanitizer, you can anticipate a renewed feeling of mental clarity. It can allow you to concentrate better and stay focused on the things that are most important at the moment. This is a great addition to any sanitizer that you play on keeping with you in your bag because it can help you stay alert while you are driving. You will learn to appreciate the calmness, yet focus, that it provides.

Tea Tree

This is a very potent oil and some people do not enjoy how strong it smells. Tea tree oil is full of benefits, though. It is one of the most highly antiseptic and antibacterial essential oils which is why it makes a lot of sense to add it to your homemade hand sanitizer recipes. As it helps you to heal from inflammation, tea tree oil can also calm you down in the same way that peppermint can. If you are able to handle the smell, this can create a very effective hand sanitizer that you will feel confident in. You will notice an overall improvement in your mood and alertness.

Rosemary

Not as commonly used, rosemary oil is great with helping your memory. When you need to retain information, smelling something that contains rosemary oil before and after can help you. It gives you a pleasant scent, but because it is not as fruity or floral as other essential oils, it is less commonly selected for hand sanitizers. Mixing a little bit of rosemary oil with lemon oil can provide you with a rejuvenating blend if you do not want to use it on its own. The rosemary oil will ensure that you are alert and ready to retain any information that comes your way.

Geranium

A floral scent that is known for being relatively mild, adding geranium oil to your sanitizer can provide you with a pleasant smell without being too overpowering. Many people who are sensitive to strong scents enjoy using geranium oil because it is subtle. It is the most floral scent of the above oils, but when used sparingly, it can give your sanitizer just enough added scent without giving you a headache. Smelling geranium on a regular basis can lift your mood, allowing you to feel happier. It may also help relieve PMS symptoms. You will feel instantly relaxed when you smell this essential oil in your homemade hand sanitizer.

Aromatherapy is very important to consider when you are crafting your own hand sanitizer recipes. The more that you familiarize yourself with the process, the better you will feel about experimenting. Making your own hand sanitizer can be a fun process that allows everyone in the family to have their own custom blend. As you can see, essential oils do a lot more for the sanitizer than adding a pleasant scent to it. These oils provide additional benefits to your hand sanitizers, and you can choose the ones more useful or appropriate for you and your family.

How Does sanitizer Work?

Sanitizer kills the microorganisms against which it is used. Disinfectant has a denaturing effect, i.e., it changes the protein structures of the microorganisms. Some disinfectants also damage the membrane of the virus or the nucleic acids of the germs. The self-made disinfectants especially aim to change the protein-containing structures due to the alcohol they contain.

Chapter 3: Gathering the Necessary Equipment

For all the recipes in this book, you'll need either a jar or small bowl for mixing your sanitizer, measuring cups and spoons, and of course a spoon (or better yet, a whisk) for stirring. (You can certainly make ·larger batches by doubling or otherwise scaling up the amounts of ingredients if you're really planning to stock up, in which case you'll need a larger bowl!) A funnel can also be useful for transferring your sanitizer to a storage container without spilling. Avoiding contamination is also an issue here – all the equipment you're going to use to make your hand sanitizer, including bowls, spoons, jars, should be thoroughly cleaned and sanitized before use. In terms of storage, most people say that old, empty pump or squirt bottles get the job done just fine. For maximum convenience, you're definitely going to want a container that can easily dispense a consistent amount of sanitizer onto your hands, because as we'll discuss later, the amount you use is actually important. Also, make sure that whatever storage option you choose is air-tight to avoid having your sanitizer evaporate or spilling. If you are recycling an old product container, though, be sure to clean it out well, including the lid, nozzle, etc. and make sure to sanitize it before filling it with your sanitizer. One easy way to do this is to spray some rubbing alcohol inside the container and let it sit until the alcohol has evaporated. Also, don't forget to label your container so that no-one accidentally ingests   your   sanitizer. Having a piece of knowledge on how to make disinfectant is excellent because you can make from natural ingredients blended with essential oils, you can quickly achieve a natural viral and antibacterial effects. This means you are a terror to germs via your own handmade disinfectant as a regular bottle of hand sanitizer is always around you.

Chapter 4: Various types of hand sanitizers

There are different types of hand sanitizers and I explained few of them which is also the common one that you can make easily from your homes and the recipes for it can be easily seen in our kitchens and farms.

One of them is the alcoholic hand sanitizer which can be made by using some alcoholic substances like, ethanol, isopropyl with other ingredients to form the sanitizer. I really prefer using isopropyl because of its qualities. It is flammable and dries the skin completely after usage. It kills germs and bacteria faster and it is also added because of its strength to fight bacteria. It is very active and effective when used to make sanitizer and a certain amount in percentage is needed to boast the strength of the sanitizer and make it work efficiently. Another type of hand sanitizer that I will discuss about again is the nonalcoholic one that involves using other ingredients like aloe vera to produce it. Aloe vera is a special leaf that is nutrient and helps in fighting diseases as well, it has other natures like nourishing the body, keeping it refreshed and smooth. It works perfectly in this type of sanitizer when mixed with other substances like glycerol and mix completely with distilled water at a certain measurement and calculations.

It stays longer on the skin unlike the alcoholic based hand sanitizer and leaves the skin with a lovely sweet smell whenever it is applied on it.

But the alcohol-based sanitizer is considered to be more effective and work faster. There are other things added to it to make it soluble and they include the glycerol that I mentioned earlier which is a simple compound that odorless and colorless in nature, very viscous liquid, nontoxic and have a very smart taste though it can be used for making food but research showed also that it may lead to some side effects like headache, vomiting and even nausea when taking into the body system. But it is really good for making of various hand sanitizer because of those qualities in it.

So, when doing the alcohol-based hand sanitizer, always have in mind that it is inflammable and can burn in blue flame when in contact with fire so it must be kept out of it. This is to help you to be cautious about it by keeping it out from it and put it away from the reach of your kids.

The spray bottle is really needed to which will serve as the final collector.it is a bottle that has a nob for spraying and its very good for the sanitizer liquid to be able to control the usage of it in an appropriate way. It is necessary to wash before using to avoid some germs and bacteria hiding in it and contaminating the solution when it is poured inside. So, for you to wash it, you will first use the distilled water to wash thoroughly and then rinse it later with the alcohol because of the bacteria and germs for alcohol has the strength of killing every germs and bacteria that might be hiding in it. This is to make sure that you are using a completely free from germs bottle so that your sanitized solution be made pure and free from any form of contaminations.

It is very portable and you can carry it whenever and where you go. There will not be any damage to the skin when you use this but the perfect work is the ability to eliminate the microorganisms. From the skin and make sure it is protected and preserved from diseases caused by germs or bacteria.

It makes the skin to look fresh.it is advisable to monitor it to avoid wrong usage by the kids or anybody who does not really know what it is so after the production, you are advised to make a label and stick on it for precautions .

We have another substance called the essential oil or tea tree oil which is also needed to make the sanitizer and this is gotten when you steam the leaves of Australia tea tree. This oil is very good antibacterial and it is used for treating so many bacteria and germ causing diseases like lice.it is very good for the hand sanitizer because of its medicinal nature.

Another material for making the sanitizer is the hydrogen peroxide which can be said to be a very good antiseptic and is used to cure some infectious diseases of the skin. This is dangerous to health when taken in or consumed by very effective to the skin for killing diseases. This material is needed in the hand sanitizer to make it work effectively.

When It's Safe to Use Hand Sanitizer—and When You Need to Find Soap and Water

Yeah, we remember, you were told about a bazillion times during the cold and flu season, to wash your hands daily. A brief refresher on why it's so, so important: Virus-containing droplets expelled through sneezes or coughs can be easily transmitted between people— even by merely shaking hands or grabbing a doorknob and then touching your nose or mouth.

So even in those cases, a wash with soap and water is your best option (after a flu shot, of course), a sink isn't always readily available; often you can't just pry yourself away from your office, whether you're in the midst of an outdoor workout. "You can't just be in the bathroom washing your hands all day," says Pritish K. Tosh, MD, a physician and researcher at the Mayo Clinic for infectious disease.

Join the sanitizer by hand. The alcohol-based gel plays the role of a knight in shining armor for those of us who can't help scrub-a-dub-dub around the clock from what we are doing. "It seems like an excellent idea to use them because of their simplicity and effectiveness," Dr. Tosh agrees.

And sometimes the hand sanitizer is a good idea — as long as you obey certain basic rules.

If soap and water are not available, disinfect your hands with a hand sanitizer Washing your hands with soap and water is always the first line of protection against a host of disease-inducing species, Dr. Tosh says. But when you can't get it to the sink, hand sanitizer will battle specific bugs too, like cold-causing viruses and flu.

Nonetheless, a report published in the journal Pediatrics this week poses concerns about conditions where a hand sanitizer can be more successful than washing up. The study showed that young children were less likely to get sick and skip daycare when they were using hand sanitizer than when they were washing their hands.

"Since the use of hand sanitizers is also convenient, people might be more likely to do it and use so more frequently than anyone would just stick to soap and water," Dr. Tosh hypothesizes. "And though the effectiveness [of hand sanitizer] may be smaller, there may be greater overall potential to avoid infection as it's easier to do more often." However, he says, experts aren't giving us the green light to fully skip the sink.

Should not use hand sanitizer when your hands are filthy. According to the Centers for Disease Control and Prevention (CDC), when your hands are coated in the muck, sanitizers actually will not function as well — say after you've been planting or tinkering with your bike gears.

For example, if you just apply sanitizer to the mix, the dirt and grease won't go anywhere, says TanayaBhowmick, MD, assistant professor of infectious disease medicine at the Robert Wood Johnson Medical School in New Jersey. "When you've got dirt on your hands and put alcohol on it, you're just making a slurry." She says you're going to rub the gunk around without ever washing it off.

And because hand sanitizer doesn't destroy every microbe, she underlines that there are those that you just need to wash off.

Ensure sure the sanitizer is at least 60% alcohol. The alcohol serves as what's considered a denaturing agent, explains Dr. Tosh, as opposed to soap, which serves as a detergent. Essentially, alcohol destroys or inactivates viruses— and, according to the CDC, it does so most efficiently in sanitizers that are between 60 and 95 percent alcohol.

Proper application, Dr. Bhowmick adds, is also essential. Apply hand sanitizer to one hand's palm, then "keep rubbing around all your hands until it's warm," she says. Pleasant reminder: You shouldn't have your hand sanitizer cleaned off, whether you're using a towel or your jeans ' legs (hey, we were there). "It defeats the intent, because whatever you wipe it off on, you may be picking up something else," says Dr. Bhowmick.

We like the vegan Instant Hand Sanitizer from Noodle & Boo ($10, dermstore.com), and the Advanced Hand Sanitizer from Purell with aloe ($13 for 4, amazon.com). It's a wise idea to look for an alcohol-based sanitizer with a moisturizing agent like aloe, Dr. Tosh says, because all that alcohol will dry up.

Avoid something branded as "antibacterial" If you're an obsessive user of hand sanitizer, you may have wondered if you're too full of it. Luckily, gels based on alcohol will continue to work just as well over time, so keep on rubbing on. "At least up to now, there's no evidence suggesting this isn't as successful [over time]," Dr. Bhowmick says — at least when it comes to killing viruses. Some research indicates that drug-resistant bacteria can develop an alcohol tolerance, though, she says.

That's a little worrying, considering the ever-growing danger of microbial resistance— when bacteria evolve to survive the antibiotics usually used to kill them. Dr. Tosh says that overuse of antibacterial and antimicrobial products will bolster those so-called superbugs, so stay away from the hand gels on their labels that advertise those properties.

Chapter 5: Five ways to make a homemade sanitizer

Gentle Hand Sanitizer Formula (Safe for Kids)

A non-drying, natural hand sanitizer gel feeds on aloe vera. It's so easy to be able to help the kids make it.

Prepare Time: 1 minute

Ingredients:

- 1/4 cup aloe vera gel
- 20 drops destroyer germ essential oil

Directions

Combine all ingredients and store in a reusable silicone container.

Stronger Hand Sanitizer Formula

Using as needed to eliminate germs naturally from Stronger Hand Sanitizer Recipe. Use this recycle for a more reliable hand sanitizer that works like commercial versions (without the triclosan). If you're operating in a hospital, this might be a perfect one for personal use. This recycle I wouldn't use on kids!

Ingredients:

- 1 TBSP rubbing alcohol
- 1/2 tsp vegetable glycerin (optional)
- 1/4 cup aloe vera gel
- 20 drops Germ Destroyer oil
- 1 TBSP distilled water or colloidal silver / ionic silver for extra antibacterial activity
- Other essential oils (just for scent)

Directions

To produce, blend aloe vera gel, optional glycerin, and rub alcohol in a small bowl.

Add essential oil of cinnamon and tea tree oil along with a drop or two of any other oils that you wish to add for fragrance. Sweet options include lemongrass, peach, lavender, and peppermint.

Mix well and add about one tablespoon of distilled water (or ionic/colloidal silver) to thin consistency if desired.

To pass hand sanitizer into a spray or pump-style bottles, using a small funnel or medicine dropper. This can also be packed for use on the go in small silicone tubes.

Using any other form of hand sanitizer as you can.

Strongest Homemade Hand Sanitizer Formula (5 Minute Formula)

To effectively kill viruses, the CDC recommends at least 60 percent alcohol in hand sanitizer. This formula follows the percentage and adds aloe vera for gentleness and essential oils for the fight against new viruses. This is the one that I'm using after working in places where the transmission of infections is more likely.

Ingredients:

- 2/3 cup alcohol rubbing (70 percent or higher)
- 2 Teaspoons aloe vera (if aloe vera can not be found, glycerin may be used as a substitute)
- 20 drops Germ Destroyer Essential Oil (You can also use Germ Fighter which is more robust, but I wouldn't recommend it for use on kids)

Directions

Mix all the ingredients and combine them in a spray bottle (these are the best size) or any small container. Use as you wish.

Keep in mind that the formula should be changed according to the strength of the alcohol you're using. For example, if you're using 99% Isopropyl rubbing alcohol, you're going to need a different amount of aloe vera than if you're using 70% alcohol. Below are some fast guidelines.

Option 1 - with 99% Isopropyl Rubbing Alcohol: two parts of alcohol and one part of aloe vera gel (e.g., 2/3 cup alcohol + 1/3 cup aloe vera gel).

Option 2 - with 91% isopropyl or rubbing alcohol: three parts whiskey and one part aloe vera gel (e.g., 3/4 cup alcohol + 1/4 cup aloe vera gel).

Option 3 - with 70% isopropyl or rubbing alcohol: nine parts of alcohol and one part of aloe vera gel.

Some people tend not to use alcohol in their hand sanitizer because alcohol has a strong odor and can have a significant drying effect on the skin.

Witch Hazel-Based Hand Sanitizer

A perfect option is the use of a witch-hazel-based sanitizer. The tea tree oil has additional antiseptic benefits.

Ingredients:

- 1 cup (preferably without additives) of pure aloe vera gel
- 1/2 teaspoons hazel 30 drops tea tree oil five drops of essential oil like lavender or peppermint Spoon Funnel Glass bottle

Directions

Stir in aloe vera water, tea tree oil, and hazel witch. To thicken it, add another spoonful of aloe vera if the mixture is too thin. Remove another spoonful of witch hazel.

If it is too thick, stir the essential oil in. Since the tea tree oil's scent is already stable, the added essential oils are simple to handle. Five or so drops are meant to be enough, but mix it in one drop at a time if you want to add more.

Funn the mixture into the receptacle. Place the funnel above the jar mouth and pour in the sanitizer for the side. Fill it up, then screw it onto the lid until ready to use it.

A tiny bottle of squirt works well if you want to take the sanitizer with you all day long.

Save the remaining sanitizer in a container with a tightly fitting lid, if you make too much for the bottle.

The One Thing That Is THE ABSOLUTE BEST Germ Destroyer on The Planet (And Is As Cheap As A Bottle Of Water)

Ok. Straightforward – that is CHLORINE. And it is very good for disinfecting the commonly used surfaces like office table, dining table, and whatever you constantly touch in your hose.

Chlorine is recommended by the World Organization of Health. It is commonly used in hospitals in emergency cases when a new pathogen appears – that is unknown until the present moment.

Thus we can also use chlorine in our and for our household. But it is very important what kind of chlorine we use. That is active chlorine or sodium hypochlorite.

What to look on when you buy disinfectant

Going on with our talk about chlorine, when you are buying a disinfectant (for surfaces), it is important that you are looking not only on the front label, but also on the back label – where it should say sodium hypochlorite (or, "active chlorine" on other products).

So, if you go to the supermarket and you buy a disinfectant on which's back label it says it contains sodium hypochlorite, then that product is good and can be used efficiently for disinfecting anything in your home – by using it according to the prospect.

How to make your own disinfectant

However, if you do not find such a disinfectant at the supermarket, then you can prepare your own at home and here is how.

You most certainly have a <u>clothes' bleach</u> product in your home. This is 100% made based on sodium hypochlorite

You should use about 0.65oz of that product to 33.8oz water. A small teaspoon for instance contains about 0.17oz of liquid.

As simple as this – and there you have your homemade house disinfectant.

Conclusion

Before entering a hospital guard or wash area, hands must be washed with soap and warm water for about twenty minutes. Handwashing eliminates around 99 percent of passing microorganisms. After that, if gloves are worn out or not, routine hygienic hand disinfection ought to take place to get rid of some succeeding transient flora and also to decrease the danger of the contamination originating out of properties that are resident.

The method of hands sanitization is of fantastic significance since the potency isn't only with all the alcohol.

In summary, hand sanitization is a significant process for employees to follow along with pharmaceutical and healthcare settings. Hand sanitization is just one of the chief procedures for preventing the spread of disease in pollution and hospitals inside pharmaceutical operations. This essential degree of control demands the usage of a successful hand sanitizer.

Printed in Great Britain
by Amazon

38114905R00023